"Finally a book to share with colleagues and patients about end-of-life decisions and plann_ _ _ _ _ _ _ _ _ _ _ _ _ _ _ st read for all patients and famili_ _ _ _ _ _ _ _ _ _ _ _ d gently guides the readers to ra_ _ _ _ _ _ _ _ _ _ _ _ 'r or Later makes it easy for pr _ _ _ _ _ _ _ _ _ _ _ y subject. With great enthusias_ 'r Later for medical, nursing and social work school curriculum to help _ _ _ _ ents gain a comfort level in dealing with real life crises_

L_ _ _ _ _ _ _ung MSN FNP, California Prison Health Care

"Sooner _ _ _ _ _ r is a courageous and well-written guide which ma_ _ _ _ _ _ ybody question how to approach one's end of life _ _ _ _ _ e and style. With so many years at the bedside, Dam_ _ _ _ _ the opportunity to witness the needless suffering and st_ _ _ _ _ _ g of many patients who pursued a plan of futile treatments. For the well and the ill, *Sooner or Later* is a breath of fresh air and an affirmation for living well, even until one's last day."

Gisele and Yvon Cariou, Yorba Linda, California

"This book is a must read for anyone looking for guidance about quality of life during its last stages. Damiano does an excellent job in helping to define and simplify end-of life-choices that we must all make. It is a reminder to me as a health care professional to help patients and their families make informed choices."

Stan Bisho RN, BSN, PHN

Thanks to Damiano's book, *Sooner or Later*,…my husband and I were able to get through four of the hardest months of our lives with our best friend, John. We both highly recommend this book to anyone with a terminal illness to better accept the future and to help families process the pain of loss. *Sooner or Later* is a must read that we think all doctors and nurses should provide to their patients."

Mr. and Mrs. Donald Visceglie, Tampa, Florida

SOONER OR LATER

RESTORING SANITY TO YOUR END-OF-LIFE CARE

DAMIANO DE SANO IOCOVOZZI, MSN FNP CNS

FOREWORD BY
MAJOR KATHLEEN WHITE, RN MS FNP

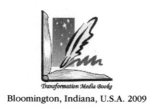

Transformation Media Books
Bloomington, Indiana, U.S.A. 2009

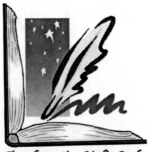

Transformation Media Books

Published by Transformation Media Books, USA
www.TransformationMediaBooks.com

An imprint of Pen & Publish, Inc.
Bloomington, Indiana
(812) 837-9226
info@PenandPublish.com

www.PenandPublish.com

www.SoonerorLaterBook.com

ISBN: 978-0-9842258-6-6

LCCN: 2010922181

This book is printed on acid free paper.

Printed in the USA

Dedication

To Thomas Walls and Drew Johnson
who teach me constantly how to live.

Table of Contents

Thanks and Gratitude

Sooner or Later has been on my mind for the last 23 years working full-time in the health care setting. I have worked as a registered nurse, clinical nurse specialist, family nurse practitioner and college lecturer over my career.

Here I would like to thank those many patients, family members and students whom I got close to during some very bad times and very good times. During those years, I believe my knowledge and skill helped my many patients find their appropriate levels of care, be it for a restoration of health or entrance into a hospice program for their final months.

To those many families and friends, thank you for letting me share those most precious moments with you.

To my parents, Vincent and Rose, and my siblings, Mary Magdalene, Cosmas, Gerry and Vincent, thank you for being my first teachers and friends. Thank you for the support, love and, humor you have given over the years.

To my maternal grandmother, Mary Terzo DiSano, thank you for showing me what was truly important from an early age. You approached life and death with grace, elegance and dignity.

To my Italian family, Maria LoRe, Ignazio LoRe and Francesca Ancona, a special thank you for all the family holidays through Italy and France. Thanks for teaching me also at an early age to live within my means and to find joy in the intangible.

A special thank you to Jeff Jones, my neighbor and his friend, Maribeth Pyne, who found me my most wonderful publisher, Ginny Weissman. If it weren't for Jeff and Maribeth, *Sooner or Later* would never have been born.

To all my neighbors and friends, thanks for the encouragement as I read *Sooner or Later* over and over to you.

Foreword

By Major Kathleen White, RN MS FNP

Over the past 100 years, demographic and historical changes have significantly altered life expectancy, the size of the population over 65 and the experience of death and dying. Advances in health promotion and medical interventions have resulted in more individuals living longer with chronic conditions and degenerative diseases. This can present individuals and families with complex and difficult decisions about medical treatment to extend life, as well as the timing and setting of the dying process.

Sooner or Later is a definitive, focused resource for individuals, their friends and families to successfully navigate medical decision making in end-of-life care. The compassionate examples and targeted lists of questions for the health care team serve to empower the seriously ill patient, and their caregivers, in their decision making toward improving the quality of life on this chapter of their journey.

The author's vast 23 years of clinical experience in advanced practice nursing, critical care and as a primary care provider brings a new and welcome approach to addressing the problems, challenges, stigma and uncertainties facing individuals and their care givers. It assists them in making informed choices about the most appropriate level of care that accommodates their needs and wishes. Through contemplation of one's mortality, an individual can begin to identify and articulate preferences that support a "good" death as described by the Congressional Research Service on End-of-Life Care, typically described as free from pain and suffering, in the company of loved ones, reflective of peace and meaning for the individual.

I am grateful for the opportunity to use this valuable resource in my clinical practice and eagerly anticipate that primary care and specialty practices, palliative and hospice care programs will consistently offer this unique tool to their clients.

Preface

I'd like to share a moment from my own childhood, which was spent growing up in an upstate New York funeral home in the Adirondacks. As a little boy, I thought everyone had a casket showroom in the basement, pretty flowers lining the walls, and occasionally a beautifully laid-out old neighbor sleeping in a highly polished piece of furniture for a few days.

My siblings and I would take fresh orchids and roses to our teachers, even in the middle of a blizzard. A neighbor's death was a serious occasion for a party; people congregated in our first-floor living room, mingling, talking, and laughing. After the burial, the crowd moved to the deceased's house for food, drinks, and more conversation. That was my life in the 1950s and 1960s.

Decades later, as a registered nurse, I see things a little differently. I still have no fear of death nor of seeing a deceased person lying in state. I certainly am not afraid to be dead. However, I am terrified of losing my independence and being sick with a loss of body control.

I'll be many things to you while reading this book: a trustworthy old friend, a doting godfather, or a battle-scarred registered nurse. Now, just call me Dom.

Introduction

"A single event can awaken within us a stranger totally unknown to us. To live is to be slowly reborn."

Antoine de Saint-Exupery

If you suffer from a life-threatening illness and are told by your health care provider (physician, physician assistant, or nurse practitioner) that you may have little chance of a medical cure or going into remission, Sooner *or Later: Restoring Sanity to Your End-of-Life Care* is my gift to you. It is written for a newly-diagnosed, terminally ill person like you or a family member, to help guide you to a place of rational decision-making. This way, you can live your life as fully as possible, and without fear.

This book also serves the loved ones of those that are terminally ill and, believe it or not, anyone who enjoys good health, and wants to live life more deeply, more in the present moment and more courageously. I want to help you and your family cope with and understand what you're facing.

For those who might be confused about the meaning of a diagnosis, this book will help you frame the important questions you need to ask your health care providers to completely understand the estimated length and quality of your lifespan.

One of my motivations for writing *Sooner or Later* is to protect you from desperate choices based on erroneous information, and the pipe dreams of an unachievable cure. I offer you my

23 years of knowledge and experience at the bedside of my patients and friends. It is my hope you will know and see where you truly stand, and understand what you can expect in the near future. I also want to help you recognize the false promise of a cure and be empowered to walk away from the temptation of pursuing one – which I call a fool's errand. My goal for you is to take control today – right now! – and remain there, sane and rational.

Try to differentiate yourself between being a patient – one who has the potential for a cure or a remission – to a pilgrim – one who can no longer achieve a cure or remission. It may help to see yourself as a pilgrim, embarking on a new journey, instead of expecting to be cured and being able to resume your old life. For a pilgrim, the way is different. No one can describe exactly what lies ahead. Every person's experience is different. However, *Sooner or Later* will empower you to remain in command, without false illusions or fear.

It is my sincere hope that this book can tell you when it's necessary to go to a Plan B or Plan C. It is written to guide you to a place of acceptance as you realize that sometime in the future, you will cease to be physically alive. Until then, use the diagnosis to create your pilgrimage of a lifetime, a road each of us must take and take alone.

Let's explore ways to use this precious time wisely. If you have exhausted every medical avenue, traditional or non-traditional, and have found yourself with no more options, *Sooner or Later* will guide you. It offers you established systems that will enable you to finish your life with control and freedom from anxiety and pain.

There are a few things *Sooner or Later* isn't. It does not attempt to answer questions from the spiritual or religious realms. I leave it to the theologians, leaders at your place of worship and philosophers to explore the bigger questions pertaining to our origins, our purpose and if there's life after death. *Sooner or Later* remains in the world of the here and now, the world of science, senses and ethics, and what I can share from my medical and nursing experience. My book is concerned with that space in your life between your diagnosis and your choice of an appropriate level of care.

Every human being has a beginning and an end. We are all fated to die one day, whether young or old, rich or poor – usually from illness, accident, or old age. It happens sooner or later. Yes, where a cure or remission is possible, by all means pursue it and keep yourself as healthy as possible. That's rational and easy. This book targets those in a "no man's land," where powerful treatments or medicines no longer work because of harm or futility. If you are unsure how to move forward or are unsure of your status due to little or no information, or a hesitant health care provider, or perhaps your own state of denial, Sooner or Later can guide you to a place of clarity.

If you don't feel you have a clear diagnosis and direction to take, use this book as your compass. It will provide you with the many questions to ask your providers so you can form a clear picture of where you are today, and how your particular case fits in ethically with the goals of medicine. Numerous, concrete examples will follow. This book will help you get the answers you seek by phrasing the questions to ask your providers during the diagnosis phase. You can use the same questions for a second and third opinion. Utilizing the answers you receive from a variety of sources, you will be better informed and able to seek the appropriate level of care.

If you are terminally ill, this book may help guide you to systems and a realistic hope that can meet your needs. This would certainly begin with the freedom to remain in your own home, surrounded by your favorite things and familiar people. You would also be free of life support machines, feeding tubes, urinary drainage bags, the hum of the intensive care unit (ICU) and a cast of characters all trying to do something *to* you, rather than *for* you.

In *Sooner or Later*, I distinguish between healing and curing. You will be empowered to make informed choices and give informed consent. You will create and take the time to make that final trip, broach topics you've eluded for years which most people refuse to talk about, and continue to grow as a unique human being until your final breath. Your new power will liberate you while allowing others to better deal with their own grief as they prepare for life without you. You give others the permission to be truthful when you accept the truth yourself. It takes a great deal of energy and effort to live in denial, pretending everything's fine, while you are really stressing out when things fall apart. It's difficult for me to see families performing these types of psychological cartwheels, nurturing false hopes while becoming more fatigued trying to live a lie. It's madness.

In my experience, most people rarely bring up the subject of death and dying, for reasons that are still unclear to me. Many seem very uncomfortable looking at a lifespan with a beginning and an end. Most people have little exposure to the very sick, most of whom are hidden from view at home, in a hospital, or in a nursing home. Few ever visit. In my daily life, I sometimes hear the same excuses to mask the discomfort: "I don't want to interrupt or disturb him." "I am uncomfortable going to a nursing home." "I want to remember her as a well person." "I don't like the smells of hospitals."

Maybe people deal with their fears by getting busier, or drowning out their fears by watching more television, cranking up the volume on their radios or iPods, or creating more cell phone ringtones to blot out uncomfortable thoughts. Perhaps thoughts of our own mortality or the eventual death of a relative, co-worker or friend provoke sufficient cause to remain distant. With knowledge that the human lifespan is so short and fleeting, wouldn't it be a welcome change to choose our words with more care, more kindness, and more respect? Wouldn't we be more compassionate knowing we share the same humanity with all who breathe the same air?

The sterile atmosphere of the hospital and clinic is deceiving; in this case, sterility implies lifelessness. There is no heartbeat. Many patients and families seem unprepared to deal with a terminal diagnosis, hospitalization, procedures and diagnostics. Some fall apart. Others find comfort in cold, clinical technology and medical terminology. Sometimes, the presentation and the reaction of the diagnosis seems divorced from any human feeling, dissected and described like a frog in science class. Do some providers, patients and families think this medical barrier can separate and shield them? Some do. To me, many providers and patients' families seem separated from their human selves, from real emotion, feelings of empathy and a commitment to be there for each other.

In times of stress, much of the human conversation in the clinic or hospital can turn highly clinical and technical, leaving the newly diagnosed person feeling more isolated and afraid. Just ask anyone confined to a nursing home or hospital room to tell you how lonely and abandoned he or she feels. *Sooner or Later* may help you sort out your feelings and feel less frightened and more in control.

During times of high stress, you may not be able to think clearly and may even consider the health care providers as minor medical deities who can fix any malady so we can get well and live happily ever after. Many providers also buy into this notion. That is, to me, magical thinking.

Sooner or Later will help facilitate a conversation between you and your significant others that most would be too terrified to start, otherwise. This is a conversation about seeing yourself as a whole person who has a beginning and an end. We can approach this the same way we may comfort a child who thinks there are monsters in his bedroom, by looking together in all the drawers, closets, and under the bed. Chances are, we will find no monsters – nothing to be afraid of!

Together, let's savor the gift of life through our senses, Let's realize that our time on this planet is not forever, but that it is ever changing, even terrifying at times, yet comforting, familiar, and beautiful. It reminds me of a quick exchange from the 1958 film *Auntie Mame,* which starred Rosalind Russell:

Auntie Mame: Oh Agnes! Here you've been taking my dictations for weeks and you haven't heard the message of my book. Live!

Agnes Gooch: Live?

Auntie Mame: Yes! Live! Life's a banquet and most poor suckers are starving to death!

Chapter One

Today Is the First Day of the Rest of Your Life

"To thine own self be true, and it must follow, as the night the day, thou canst not then be false to any man."

William Shakespeare, *Hamlet*

Sooner or Later is a manual for seekers, for people facing a life-threatening illness, as well as their family and friends. It's for people seeking calm and sanity in a topsy-turvy situation. Since relatively few talk about the path that leads out of this life, I will talk about it here. Consider me your tour guide, one who knows a thing or two about these particular passages.

In my twenty-three year career as a registered nurse, clinical nurse specialist, and family nurse practitioner, I have experienced things most people cannot imagine. I have been with people through their best and worst of times: people including patients, friends, family members, and my spouse.

1

I have held people while they suffered through terrible pain and grief. I've laughed with them during a triumph, bathed and fed them, medicated them ... and even caught a baby who entered the world in a parked car! I have also had the privilege of being present during the sacrament of a person's last breaths, holding their hand for the last time, and closing their eyes as tears formed in my own.

As a nurse living at the edge of life and everywhere in between, my gift to you is a rich distillation of bedside wisdom to help guide you through some rough, crazy patches from which no living being is immune and for which few are prepared. We learn a lot about how to earn a living, keep a job and raise children, but who teaches us how to manage our own health care? Who teaches us that we have power beyond measure? Who teaches us how to finish our lifespan with richness, grace, and control? Who teaches us how to live each moment, like Auntie Mame proclaims?

The precious time between diagnosis and your last day can and should be special. Your last months of life should be devoted to doing what's most important to you: preparing your way, letting go of anger and sorrow, finishing your life's business, enjoying yourself, making amends and creating lasting memories for those you must leave behind. For all your large and small responsibilities, you will find time and energy to have fun, visit and laugh. Many tell me that during this time, they have never felt so alive and free. Artificial barriers and pretenses to real emotions may be lifted as our human communication becomes more honest, poignant and sane. For some, it is a gracious time, a time of generosity and passing on a legacy, an appropriate climax for a life well-lived. Couldn't we all live in such a space, even if we are not facing a life-threatening illness? *Sooner or Later* may take you on a journey of self-discovery, empower you to remain in control and have your wishes honored.

In her book *Return to Love: Reflections on the Principles of A Course in Miracles,* Marianne Williamson writes, "Our deepest fear is not that we are inadequate. Our deepest fear is that we are powerful beyond measure. It is our light, not our darkness that most frightens us. We ask ourselves, Who am I to be brilliant, gorgeous, talented, fabulous? Actually, who are you not to be? You are a child of God. Your playing small does not serve the world. There is nothing enlightened about shrinking so that other people won't feel insecure around you. We are all meant to shine, as children do. We were born to make manifest the glory of God that is within us; it's in everyone. And as we let our own light shine, we unconsciously give other people permission to do the same. As we are liberated from our own fear, our presence automatically liberates others."

That liberation begins with the liberation of good knowledge. Where can you find honest, scientific information about your condition that is personal to you? Your health care providers (physician, physician assistant, nurse practitioner) are your best sources. In addition, registered nurses or social workers are excellent resources. Interview a variety of them during a family conference. If the answers you receive from these trained, empathetic professionals are basically the same, you're there. The Internet and your public library can help you obtain research articles, pharmaceutical information and even information about ethics, hospice and palliative care.

The next few chapters will help put you in an ethical framework, see the appropriate medical goals for yourself, fill out an Advance Health Care Directive (AHCD) and obtain additional information about hospice and palliative care.

Chapter Two

Say What You Mean and Mean What You Say

"Saint Francis of Assisi was hoeing his garden when someone asked him what he would do if he were suddenly informed that he would die before sunset that very day. 'I would finish hoeing my garden,' he replied."

Anonymous

This chapter begins the nuts-and-bolts discovery of where you stand on the continuum of your lifespan and how to maximize your remaining time. It starts with an emotional assessment and offers words and meaning to the rollercoaster ride of emotions you may be experiencing right now. During this discovery process, please permit yourself to be strong and never let anyone hobble or disable your pursuit of finding out exactly where you are, even if it's out of love. When you are obtaining medical opinions from your providers or specialists, take this book with you to their offices. Use the questions provided to cut to the chase and even write out questions that are pertinent and specific to your situation and how you feel. Take one or two people with you to listen intently and jot down the answers.

Before beginning the work of organizing family conferences with your current or potential providers, let's do an emotional self-assessment. This will enable you and your significant others to look at the stages of grief that accompany bad news. In 1969, Dr. Elisabeth Kubler-Ross wrote a landmark book called *On Death and Dying*, which millions of patients, family members and friends have since found to be an invaluable resource. It might serve you in the same way.

Dr. Kubler-Ross breaks down grief into five stages that unfold like this: upon receipt of some very bad news, our emotions run a gamut that begins with denial, dives into anger and shifts to bargaining before experiencing depression, and eventual acceptance. Usually nobody stays for long in one of those stages, but moves back and forth between all the stages. It is a very fluid process in which stages can change by the day – or sometimes, by the minute. Over a period, the shock becomes less severe and we, as adaptable human beings, can finally accept the news.

Use these next questions to help moor yourself in a safe harbor in your mind. Sort out your emotions to remain rational and make sound decisions.

The Self Assessment (Write your answers in the spaces)

1. How am I feeling emotionally now?

2. What stage of grief am I experiencing right now? Shock? Anger? Denial?

3. Am I bargaining with God to give me more time? Am I depressed?

4. Did I hear anything the providers or specialists told me?

5. How are my significant others dealing with this bad news?

6. What remaining personal goals do I still need to accomplish?

7. Who are the people I have harmed during my lifetime? Who are the people who have harmed me?

8. From whom must I seek forgiveness? Whom must I forgive?

9. How can I deal with my fears of death?

10. Who can I trust to speak for me if I'm no longer able?

11. How can I be assured others will honor my wishes?

12. What would I like to do for myself or others that would give me great pleasure?

13. What preparations must I make for myself and others?

14. What must I do to finally accept what has happened to me?

Let's assume you have held a family conference with your provider or a specialist, and that person has given you some very bad news. Let's conduct a review and turn over every stone that leads from then until now. Let's make sure you are clear on the information you've been given by your providers. Let's continue with another series of questions. Use this section as a workbook and fill in your answers in the spaces provided.

1. If you found that your health has changed, did all of your tests, labs, physical examinations and consultations provide a verifiable scientific diagnosis?

2. Did you obtain a second or a third opinion? If not, will you do so now?

3. Did your providers offer any indication there was a cure?

4. Did you weigh your options if all those opinions were the same? What if the opinions differed? What will you do now?

5. Did you attempt a cure?

6. Were you cured?

7. Is the disease worsening now? Did it return?

   If you still are uncertain about your diagnosis or path forward, or if the disease has come back or worsened to a point that is now threatening your life, let's continue to explore where you go from here. If a diagnosis was made and you have no further ability to be cured or be in remission, today is the day to take control of the rest of your life!

The Agendas

   All kinds of agendas will surface where you least expect them, especially after a bonafide terminal diagnosis is given. These are agendas that could possibly take you on a fool's errand when you may be unwilling. Some family members may push you to try every possible cure or treatment if they depend on your income to pay their bills. If you and your significant others have unresolved emotional or family issues, both you and they may think you need more time to work on those – or, unfortunately, remain in denial about them. Your health care provider may even suggest treatments that many may believe are futile.

There are all kinds of agendas to consider; more will pop up unexpectedly. Just bear this in mind: The whole process will be colored by your own feelings and agendas, and the agendas of your significant others. Things can and will become very complicated if you end up trying to please everybody else and not yourself.

In the end, it is your life and your decision. Empower yourself to stay in control and lead your family to a place that is appropriate for you. Eventually, your loved ones may see it your way. Empower them to feel grief, to go through its stages, to take action to prepare themselves for your absence in their life, perhaps by getting a job or acquiring new job skills if they depend on your income. It is a time of personal growth for them and for you, so let it unfold.

Like all major life changes such as birth, marriage, divorce and illness, families become unsettled and sometimes unhinged when death comes knocking. As you become more settled and serene, so will your significant others; they will follow your lead. Teach them to live on, give them better coping mechanisms, and show them how to accept the human condition.

The Cast of Characters

Until proven otherwise, consider your providers to be on your side. Look at everybody you're meeting, their roles and points of view. Let's start by reviewing the professional medical model to see what motivates and guides physicians. Take a hard look at what medicine is and isn't, and later study the six medical goals in light of your illness. Let's see really where medicine can reach, and where it cannot extend.

Medicine attempts to prevent disease. When disease does occur, medicine attempts to cure it. If a disease cannot be cured, medicine tries to soften its effects or "palliate" it. Let's take arthritis. No one can cure arthritis, but you can use medicines and physical therapy, practice stretching exercises and yoga, stay warm, move to a warmer climate or find other proven means to alleviate the pain. That is palliation.

Medicine is based on the scientific method of trial and error. The "one size fits all," cookie cutter-type medicine is not ideal. All visits should be tailored to you and your individual needs and concerns. One goal of medicine is to help you live longer and with a high quality of life, whenever possible. Medicine cannot stop death, nor should it. Good providers recognize their own limitations and know medicine's frontier, where it can go and where its effectiveness diminishes or stops.

The old school of physicians lived in the *Father Knows Best* era. Patients were neither empowered to ask questions nor to guide their own care. Instead, they trusted their fate to the wise, old family doctor who probably delivered them. He was a respected and venerated community member whose advice was sought for medical and non-medical problems alike. No doubt he enjoyed his celebrity status in his town or city. Those days are mostly gone.

The new school of physicians is a lot different, although you get the occasional throwback to yesteryear. The newer physicians are educated to include the patient in the plan of care. Patients are respected enough to give informed consent and make up their own minds without coercion and to act autonomously. The new school physician provides guidance, information and sometimes even a sympathetic ear. Most modern physicians realize their own limitations; many have enough integrity and self-confidence to tell you, "I don't know."

Let's look at the professional nursing model and how it differs from the medical model. Registered nursing grew from Florence Nightingale's time, the mid and late 19th Century, and developed separately from the professional physician's model. Time, customs, and laws have made their functions interdependent. Nursing incorporates the medical disease-focused and primary prevention model into a larger, more holistic framework. Registered nurses view and consider the whole experience of the person, from cradle to grave. Our diagnoses also reflect the human being's place in society. We include diagnoses that reflect the psychosocial and spiritual sides. When there is no cure, the professional registered nurse has a plan to provide every comfort measure that is realistic and possible. We do not abandon the very sick, but advocate to obtain appropriate medications and comfort care. We provide support through the lifespan, through cure and palliation until the time of passing. Usually, nurses accompany you from the opening of the gate of life to its closing. Healing and comfort care always occur during this period.

In 1973, a prominent Colorado physician, Dr. Henry Silver, evolved the nurse practitioner from nursing. The nurse practitioner is a registered nurse with advanced degrees that can include Ph.D. The nurse practitioner role is different in every state, per respective regulations. The nurse practitioner shares the same general duties as physicians, including seeing patients, assessing, diagnosing, ordering appropriate tests and labs, providing treatments, and evaluating the plan of care. In some states, the nurse practitioner collaborates with physicians; in other states, the nurse practitioner can bill and operate without a physician.

Some nurse practitioners are hospitalists and see patients throughout the hospital stay, while others have privileges to admit, discharge and follow-up with the patient in the clinic. In most states, nurse practitioners can prescribe the same pharmaceuticals as physicians, including narcotics like morphine or Demerol. In some places, patients rarely see family practice physicians, as the ranks of family physicians have dwindled in numbers. Instead, they visit nurse practitioners, who are often reimbursed at the same rates as physicians for the same types of services. Ideally, both physician and nurse practitioner work for the patient, without one-upmanship. Both adequately treat patients in the primary care clinic.

By knowing the roles of physicians, registered nurses and nurse practitioners, you are now better equipped to deal with the characters you'll meet in those foreign places like hospitals, clinics, or nursing homes. Slowly, you are also learning a foreign language: medicalese. You are learning to communicate in order to receive the best options available for your particular problem. Hopefully, this will melt away confusion and fear.

Chapter Three

Medical Goals, Ethics and You

"If you want to build a ship, don't drum up people to collect wood and don't assign them tasks and work, but rather teach them to long for the endless immensity of the sea."

Antoine de Saint-Exupery

Ethics offers a moral take on human behavior. Biomedical ethics addresses behavior in a medical setting. In Chapter One, we briefly visited the goals of medicine. Let's look at them here in more depth. While this chapter may seem a little heavy at times, I've salted and peppered it with examples to make it more interesting.

The best authors to mention here are Jonsen, Siegler and Winslade, whose book, *Clinical Ethics* (1986) occupies a pocket in my lab coat to this day! The ease of how they frame complex ethical problems continues to amaze me after all these years. Since I liked their work so well, I decided to share it with you in this section because it offers considerable clarity on what you're going through. And that's what we need right now:

clarity, sanity, calmness and lots of sunlight. I'll use their framework to illustrate examples and patient pictures that come from my experience.

The goal of this chapter is to guide you through the six important goals of medicine, and then to look at some patients and place them in an ethical model. When fortified with these forms of diseases and your personal and realistic goals of medicine, it will be more difficult for you to jump on the merry-go-round of a fool's errand.

The Generic Medical Goals

1. Restoration of health

With accurate and systematic assessments, labs, diagnostic tests and your provider's experience, a verifiable diagnosis can be made regarding your particular condition. With that method, most other providers could come up with the same conclusions. Where possible, with the correct medical plan of surgery, treatment or medicine, the patient may be cured by the provider.

Example: Murray is experiencing terrible abdominal pain after eating a greasy meal. He goes to the emergency care center, is given an ultrasound and is diagnosed with an acute gallbladder, thickened walls, sludge and stones. A surgeon performs an intake and Murray is wheeled into the operating room later that day; the gallbladder is removed without complications. Murray goes home in a few days and soon returns to work.

2. Saving or prolonging a life.

Example: Amber, age 12, is involved in a terrible accident with her mother. She is not restrained in the back seat and is thrown out the window. The paramedics arrive on the scene, assess the girl and begin cardiopulmonary resuscitation (CPR) and advanced cardiac life support (ACLS). A tube is inserted into Amber's mouth and a paramedic uses a device to breathe for her. Another paramedic begins chest compressions. Amber's heart rhythm returns, but she is still not breathing on her own. She is quickly transported to the closest trauma center, where a team is waiting for her. She has emergency surgery, is stabilized and recovers in a rehab center after a few months.

Example: Ben, age 69, experiences difficulty urinating. A few blood tests are conducted, including a prostate-specific antigen (PSA) and a digital rectal exam (DRE). Later, a urologist diagnoses early prostate cancer after performing other diagnostic tests. Ben receives the appropriate treatment and now urinates without difficulty. For now, the cancer is gone. It may or may not return, so he follows up every three months.

3. Education and advice about diagnoses.

Example: Martha, age 39, has non-insulin dependent diabetes. She is taking oral medicines daily, but doesn't have a blood sugar machine for home testing. We give her a machine and teach her how to use it before breakfast. I explain the acceptable range of blood sugars she should have in the morning – between 60 and 100. I advise her to write the numbers down each morning in a small booklet. After two weeks, Martha returns and I adjust the dosages of her diabetes medicines. I instruct her to write them down every morning and return in a month to see if the adjustments have brought her sugar to an acceptable range. I give her diet and exercise handouts and arrange a consult with a dietician.

4. Hippocrates' advice to physicians, "First, do no harm!"

Example: Tony, age 52, has incurable lung cancer that spreads to his bones and liver. The cancer in his bones causes them to break and keeps him in a state of constant misery. He asks me to give him a lethal dose to kill him. I assess his feelings of helplessness and hopelessness and refer him to our local hospice care center. Later that week, I visit him in a hospice care unit nearby and see a different man who is no longer in excruciating pain. I talk with him while he smokes outside; he says he can live with the pain now. He thanks me.

5. Relief of symptoms.

Example: Dolores, 29, was involved in a bad car accident. She is experiencing pain in the neck and lower back. She was not treated in the emergency department. I assess her, order some x-rays, and send her to physical therapy. She returns two weeks later, feeling a lot better. During her initial visit, I gave her a muscle relaxant, an anti-inflammatory and a mild narcotic, which she still takes from time to time. She is ready to return to work.

6. Restoration of function or restoring some function.

Example: Doris, age 67, had a stroke recently that left her left side paralyzed; she could no longer walk. She is motivated not to lose her independence and wants to be able to lift herself in and out of a wheelchair, to the toilet, bed and car. She also wants to use a walker, if possible. Some feeling is now returning to her left side. I refer her to physical and occupational therapy. After a month, there are noted improvements: she can transfer herself from the wheelchair to her car, toilet and bed. She's working very hard to stand alone, using a walker.

Medical Goals and Forms of Disease

Let's examine three broad categories or forms of disease with the framework of these medical goals. The following are real people I had the privilege of treating. Following each patient description, I will use Jonsen, Siegler and Winslade's disease framework and note any ethical problems with each. I will discuss the medical goals which may change as the disease process advances. You may see your own particular case unfolding in a category and your personal medical goals, too.

These frameworks and the discussion that follows can show you the ethical dilemmas that may arise if you are not treated according to your unique form of disease with corresponding, realistic and attainable medical goals. Any mismatch may cause undue suffering for you, and may steer you toward a crazy fool's errand. The patient scenarios range from simple and straightforward to more complicated and ethically sensitive.

Patient One: Peter

Peter is a 24-year-old perfectly healthy young man who arrives in the emergency department with lower abdominal pain that will not go away with antacids and a bowel movement. The pain began the night before with a meal of beef, mashed potatoes, gravy and green beans. He also consumed three glasses of beer. I received Peter at the start of my shift, and conducted a physical assessment along with a few labs and ultrasound. I diagnosed him with acute appendicitis and phoned the surgeon on call; he admitted Peter and operated. The emergency appendectomy was performed without complication. Peter stayed a couple of days in the hospital and then went home.

First Form of Disease and the Goals of Medicine ACURE (acute, critical, unexpected, responsive, easily diagnosed and treated)

Peter's acute appendicitis fits well with this form of disease and meets the criteria of ACURE. He fulfilled all the medical goals discussed in this chapter. His health was restored, his symptoms went away except for the pain at the surgical site and his life was saved. He received education about how to care for the surgical site and when to follow up at the surgeon's office to remove the sutures.

Peter benefited from the surgeon's skill, sterile technique and good nursing care; no harm came to him. Peter's case was simple; ACURE rarely produces any ethical dilemmas. Peter met the medical goals for the ACURE form of disease. If things had gone wrong for Peter, for example his heart suddenly changed rhythm or if he had respiratory difficulties, failure or arrest, CPR (cardiopulmonary resuscitation), ACLS (advanced cardiac life support), and a life support machine would be appropriate for this form of disease category, as death was not expected in one previously so healthy.

Patient Two: Wanda

Wanda, age 42, is a Type 2 non-insulin dependent diabetic who was diagnosed with diabetes at age 30 when her weight jumped from 125 pounds to 225 pounds after the birth of twins. Her parents on both sides suffer from obesity; diabetes also runs among some of her aunts, uncles, and grandparents. Currently, Wanda is obese with borderline diabetes and is controlling it through diet, rather than medicine. She was previously prescribed two pills every morning, but as Wanda lost weight, improved her diet and started to exercise, we were able to discontinue the medication. Now at 199 pounds, Wanda remains a diabetic, but takes good care of herself, exercises, eats wholesome foods three times a day, comes to the clinic four times a year and gets her labs on a regular basis. Wanda visits an ophthalmologist annually and I check her feet at every visit.

Every day, she tests her own blood sugar and writes it down in a booklet I provided. She maintains an average fasting blood sugar level between 60 and 110. Wanda feels well on her routine, holds a job, raises her children and exercises twice a week with her husband. Some of our mutual goals have changed now as we're focusing on weight loss. She admits she still dreams of all things chocolate: pies, cakes and candies.

Second Form of Disease and the Goals of Medicine: COPE (chronic, out-patient, palliative [softened], efficacious [able to do something about it])

Patients in the COPE form of disease are the majority of patients seen in small primary care clinics. Wanda meets the criteria of the COPE patient: her well-controlled diabetes is chronic; she has never been hospitalized except for childbirth; the effects of diabetes are controlled by good primary care, diet, exercise, quarterly labs, foot exams, and annual eye exams. Diabetes combines four diseases into one: neurological, metabolic, kidney and cardiac. We make sure to look at all four places on each visit.

The ophthalmologist (eye physician) dilates her eyes yearly and photographs the retinas to keep blindness away; I look for foot skin breakdown, ulcers, fungus and assess sensation. To date she has no neuropathy or painful, burning feet or loss of sensation. We check her urine for large and small protein molecules, because damaged kidneys allow these molecules to pass out of the body. With quarterly labs, we check any metabolic effects the sugar may be causing, including her cholesterol and other heart plaque-forming fats. Her percentage of sugar in one red blood cell is at a pre-diabetic level (HgbA1C).

The diabetes described here is a lot like other COPE illnesses: high blood pressure, high cholesterol, asthma, arthritis and some forms of cancer. In the next chapter, I will list major diseases grouped by form of disease.

In Wanda's COPE form of disease, the primary care provider manages any end-organ damage in the kidneys, eyes and heart, any large and small vessel damage like plaque formation in the heart and the retinas of the eyes. If these effects are not monitored, the effects of diabetes progress to blindness, amputation, kidney dialysis and even heart attack.

Diabetes is a lot like that saying about a little girl. "When she's good, she's very, very good. When she's bad, she's horrid." Because of her good daily routine, Wanda remains out of the hospital and emergency room. Her care and medicines are very affordable, considering Wanda is uninsured. She's actively involved in her care, its direction and outcomes and states she's satisfied with her quality of life. There are rarely ethical dilemmas for the stable COPE patient.

However, should something change for Wanda, her heart rhythm fluctuate or another disease arrives on top of the diabetes, she may progress to the next form of disease, CARE. If Wanda experienced a change in heart rhythm or problems breathing for any reason which threatened her life, CPR and ACLS resuscitation would be appropriate for her as death was not expected in someone so healthy.

Patient Three: Edwin

The following is another true story which illustrates how a patient can go from a COPE to a CARE patient in a short time. I saw Edwin, age 40, in a primary care clinic in the San Francisco Bay Area. Edwin routinely came to see me for the occasional sore throat, cough and cold, but this visit was different. He arrived with a small, apricot-sized lump under his left arm; it protruded from beneath his shirt. Apparently, he felt the lump a few weeks previously during a business trip in Germany; at that time, it was only the size of a grape. The lump was not filled with liquid or pus, but was painless, non-moveable and somewhat hard, which was cause for worry.

Edwin was an accomplished researcher who helped develop coatings for surgical scalpels and traveled a lot. He was extremely likeable, charismatic, well-spoken and caring. Edwin could turn a room of strangers into admirers after a few minutes. He wooed all the staff in a very short time, including the providers.

During the visit, I ordered several labs including tumor markers, HIV and acute hepatitis. I also scheduled a biopsy appointment for the following week with a colleague. Since Edwin had good insurance and we were associated with a major teaching hospital, I believed he would get the best care possible. A few days after the biopsy, the pathologist called to say Edwin's lump was a non-Hodgkin's lymphoma, a rarely fatal cancer of the lymph nodes easily treated with chemotherapy and radiation. In a short time, the blood work arrived by fax.

Edwin was HIV positive and had contracted hepatitis C. Now he had a real diagnosis of AIDS (acquired immunodeficiency syndrome) that was complicated by the hepatitis C. That was very sad news for me. My personal response was physical: I experienced a bad bellyache as I informed our medical director. I later met with Edwin, who was on pins and needles since the biopsy. He still looked great, the picture of health. Edwin soon saw a colleague of mine, an oncologist who also was a noted AIDS provider.

When he returned to see me, he had a venous access device (VAD) under the skin of his chest wall to deliver the chemotherapy and to take blood samples so his arms wouldn't be stuck with needles. In addition to seeing the oncologist/AIDS specialist, Edwin sometimes returned to see me. He started to look thinner and was balding, but he was still the same old Edwin. My reports said the cancer was gone, with no other tumor sites found anywhere in the body. We were both very pleased.

Five years passed. I saw Edwin very infrequently, as he was basically managed by the oncologist/AIDS physician. One day, he returned with a different problem: abdominal pain. I ran all the usual tests and felt the liver, which was large and very painful, especially when I pressed on the gallbladder. An ultrasound confirmed a thickened gallbladder with lots of stones. Edwin had the gallbladder removed; the operating and biopsy report also noted an enlarged liver and advanced cirrhosis which was due to the hepatitis C. The labs showed an altered liver function, high bilirubin levels and very low platelets.

Additionally, the surgical incision site wouldn't heal itself. He slowly began to heal after I sent him to a registered nurse who was a wound specialist. For now, Edwin was medically stable as the wound began to heal, but he lost his sparkle. He wasn't a candidate for a liver transplant due to the AIDS and non-Hodgkin's lymphoma history.

After seeing the liver specialist, Edwin returned to see me and we discussed getting an Advance Health Care Directive (AHCD). He agreed that he was feeling worse and understood that he couldn't get a new liver. Edwin filled out the AHCD, making himself a "no code" or "do not resuscitate" patient. The following week, Edwin left for Florence, Italy to give a lecture for some European disposable instruments manufacturers. I told him to make an appointment to see me when he got back.

After he returned from Italy, I noticed that Edwin's thinking was slightly off, although he was taking medicines to ward off altered thought process. I also noticed yellowed skin and water in the abdomen. During a physical exam, I saw his eye whites were looking more yellowish and his skin a little bronzed. After that day, the liver physician basically took over. A few weeks later, the liver specialist's clerk called to say our mutual patient, Edwin, had died at home with hospice after lapsing into a coma.

Third Form of Disease and the Goals of Medicine: CARE (critical, active, recalcitrant [stubborn], eventual)

Edwin began as a COPE patient even after being diagnosed with AIDS, non-Hodgkin's lymphoma and hepatitis C. Thanks to chemotherapy, radiation and good HIV/AIDS medications, Edwin lasted for about six years in the COPE form of disease.

The one and only time he was hospitalized was to remove the gallbladder. He didn't die in a hospital nor a nursing home, but rather in his own home, surrounded by family in a hospice program. Unfortunately, after the gallbladder was removed, Edwin's condition deteriorated. I moved him from a COPE patient to a CARE patient to alleviate any ethical dilemmas and to prevent him from embarking on a futile fool's errand. None of my colleagues would have permitted that, either. Can you imagine the tragedy for Edwin if his providers still considered him as patient who could benefit from a cure or had the potential for remission?

For someone like Edwin, who was in the medical business, it was easy to level with him and steer him away from false choices and promises. Let's look more closely at the appropriate goals of medicine and how they changed because of his deteriorating liver. Although the cancer never returned and the HIV/AIDS was controlled, Edwin's sick liver created havoc with his healing process and his ability to clot. The surgical wound couldn't heal properly because his platelet count was so low. His ability to coagulate the blood to form a scab became altered. The liver has so many functions that we cannot effectively live without one.

Let's review the changing medical goals for Edwin as the liver deteriorated. After the gallbladder surgery, the hepatitis C remained at a critical point – active and recalcitrant. It would eventually cause Edwin's death. To temporarily extend his life on life support in an intensive care unit would have been an exercise in futility. What would CPR and ACLS have done for this patient? In my opinion, it would have only postponed a peaceful death. Since Edwin could not receive a new liver, the only possible medical goals for his last week of life were to relieve pain and suffering and cause no harm.

Patient Four: Drew

Drew, age 51, was new to a cardiology practice in a community hospital where I worked. Two days a week, I saw the cardiologist's patients in the hospital, admitting and discharging and then following up in the clinic. The cardiologist worked mostly in the cardiac catheterization lab, performing procedures.

Drew was a tradesman with a good job until his first heart attack. He had a smoking history, suffered from late emphysema and was obese. He had a history of sleep apnea, and used a mask and CPAP machine at night to keep his lungs inflated. I rarely saw him in clinic, but during a hospital stay, I called on him and got to know him better. His present issue was a lowered blood oxygen level, which is a chronic problem with smokers and emphysema. Usually, the body is able to compensate for the lower oxygenation.

My plan for Drew was to send him to a skilled nursing facility or home with a low-flow oxygen tank for use during the day. I also wanted to send him home with a respiratory therapist to add oxygen to his CPAP machine for night use.

It didn't happen as I suggested. Drew was still in the hospital the next time I returned to call on patients. His slim chart was now thickening with more tests, consultants' notes and even more diagnostics. Drew was looking worse and becoming depressed. From the stress of the prolonged hospitalization, he developed a stomach ulcer and later had an exploratory laparoscopy. As the weeks passed, Drew started to get infections of the lung and skin, requiring heavy antibiotics.

Shortly thereafter, Drew was on a life support machine, unconscious from heavy sedation. About a week before he died, Drew's time was consumed with more diagnostics. At one point, I asked the cardiologist if he did not see a dying man in the unit. In the team notes, I read about new plans for Drew. I wrote my own note, asking everybody on the team to agree to involve the biomedical ethics committee.

On my next visit, I found Drew to have fixed and dilated pupils, a sign of brain death. I phoned the cardiologist to tell him the situation. Later, Drew's sister was located and directed the team to turn off the life support machine. In a short time, Drew's heart stopped.

Drew's case was unfortunate, but the team certainly tried. As time passed with a prolonged hospital stay and surgery, nosocomial or hospital-borne infections set in, causing him to worsen. What medical goals were accomplished for Drew? I can only think of one, prolonging his life but at a very large personal cost to Drew.

Chapter Four

Patient Preferences, Quality of Life and Socioeconomic Factors

"For attractive lips, speak words of kindness.
For lovely eyes, seek out the good in people.
For poise, walk with the knowledge
that you never walk alone.
People, even more than things, have to be
restored, renewed and redeemed.
Never throw out anyone.
Remember, if you ever need a helping hand,
you will find one at the end of each arm.
As you grow older, you will discover that you
have two hands, one for helping yourself
and one for helping others."

Audrey Hepburn

The nuts and bolts of sound medical decision-making rest on the foundation of your wishes, autonomy, perceived quality of life and socioeconomic factors. Again, I'll call on Jonsen, Siegler, and Winslade's framework for this discussion. We'll use their framework and my examples to help you make sound decisions.

In order for your choices to be honored, the provider must deem you capable or competent to make them. In addition, providers must protect those deemed incompetent from making the wrong choices. Your mental ability must also show you can process information. Highly emotional, depressed or anxious people may demonstrate impaired judgment.

Let me provide a few examples to illustrate this point.

Example 1: Carlos, age 80, comes to see me in a new state of confusion. He is pleasant enough, but definitely confused. The previous day, he was fine, totally alert, awake and oriented. This time, he doesn't seem to know where he is, and appears a bit altered. On this day, he is totally incompetent to make any medical decision, so I leave that to his daughter. I ask him for a urine sample, test it and find he's got a new urinary tract infection, probably the reason for the altered mental state. I write a prescription and call his daughter the next day. Carlos is better: He remembers the year and the month.

Example 2: Kate, age 73, has progressive dementia, similar to the kind her mother had at Kate's age. Kate's daughter cares for her in her home. Since my suggestion, Kate now has a job: she cuts out coupons from every magazine and newspaper available and seems to be thriving with the new occupation. She lives back in the days of her youth when her children were small. Kate thinks her daughter is really Kate's deceased sister, Marge. Kate is totally incapable of making her own health care choices.

Example 3: Lucy, age 62, has a malignant thyroid nodule and has scheduled an appointment for the following week to remove it. It is very small, with no local spread. She arrives upset and tells me she cancelled her surgery. I dig deeper and find a very depressed, anxious woman who believes she would be better off dead. She has no plan to kill herself, but wants this cancer to spread so it can facilitate her death. I find a therapist that works with her for the depression, and she starts on a low dose anti-depressant. In two weeks, she has the surgery without complications. I visit with her post-operatively and she says she made the right choice. The nodule and surrounding tissue are removed. She follows up with the oncologist.

Informed Consent

As providers, we are obligated to give you the information you need to make informed decisions that will be honored. You must be informed of the risks, benefits and alternatives to what the provider is recommending. Your consent is necessary for procedures that range from a simple thing like botox injections to an appendectomy. Informed consent is much more than signing a paper. True informed consent occurs when the relationship between the provider and patient is open, honest, and respectful. It revolves around your wishes, your competence and honoring your unpressured decisions. Of course, there will always be complications like fear, anxiety and distractions on the parts of both provider and patient. If you have a life-threatening illness, you have a need to listen, to trust others and process information about the rest of your life. Remember, you are in charge!

Burdens and Benefits

Words like "ordinary" and "extraordinary" are often tossed about in living wills and Advance Health Care Directives (AHCD). "Ordinary" measures are items like food, water, nursing care, medicines, pain killers, dialysis and IV's. "Ordinary" means treating common, easily diagnosed ailments like infection, high blood sugar or a wound. They are effective, short-term, low-cost solutions that make the patient feel better quickly. The outcomes are predictable and of high benefit in the short-term.

"Extraordinary" measures comprise those things that can cause excessive pain, suffering, inconvenience or are just too costly to be of any benefit. In patients with a life-threatening illness who have no potential for cure or remission, these types of measures are universally considered futile. If you have determined yourself to be a CARE patient whose disease is progressive, incurable and stubborn, you can ask the following questions of those who are offering you new treatments that you suspect may be of no benefit or futile. You can determine if these extraordinary measures are really unnecessary from the various opinions you are receiving from family conferences.

Use the following questions to find out if your suspicions are correct or incorrect:

1. Who will benefit from this treatment or procedure? You? Me?

2. Will this test you are proposing tell you something you already know? Something you don't know?

3. How will the information from this test affect the course of my illness?

4. What new treatments will benefit me? Are these experimental?

5. In the long-term, of what benefit would any of what you are suggesting be to me?

6. What will happen to my present quality of life to do what you propose?

7. I am probably already very advanced with this life-threatening illness and do not want to spend large amounts of time grasping at straws and wasting my good days. If you were in my shoes, would you do what you are suggesting?

8. Is what you suggest futile in my case?

9. Would you put your father or mother through what you're proposing?

Some of the questions may sound similar, but the answers could be very different. Choose those questions carefully, and then add your own. Questions like those above will help you determine if what is being proposed is worthy of further consideration. If the answers are truly "extraordinary," suggest more burden than benefit, can potentially shorten your life or subtract from your quality of life, then simply walk away.

Quality of Life

First and foremost, Hippocrates instructed physicians to first do no harm. Notable goals of medicine include the improvement of the quality of life, relief of pain and suffering, supportive care, psychosocial care, and all the appropriate care for your particular form of disease: ACURE, COPE or CARE. Each form of disease helps tailor the six goals of medicine realistically for each person's case.

Your quality of life is purely what you say it is, for nobody can step into your shoes and feel exactly as you. From many patients, I often hear similar comments about their perceived quality of life. "I have more good days than bad days. Overall, I'm doing okay. I'm living at home and I try to do things for myself. That's really good for me."

Observers also comment on their significant other's quality of life. "She seems to be in no pain and comfortable." "She likes to watch her TV programs and walks about the house like before." "She seems to enjoy herself and the children more."

Socioeconomic Factors

Since we're living in a time of increasing scarcity, many people will have to pitch in and help take care of friends and family members, like in the old days. For some, visiting nurses may not be affordable, as many agencies do not take certain insurances. Even the uninsured may have difficulty getting services for a loved one without money to pay. Now everyone is vulnerable to the uncertainties of the financial world and government.

The situation reminds me of a quote attributed to our nation's sixth president: "On his eightieth birthday, John Quincy Adams responded to a query concerning his well-being by saying, 'John Quincy Adams is well. But the house he lives in at present is becoming dilapidated. It is tottering on its foundations. Time and the seasons have nearly destroyed it. Its roof is pretty well worn out. Its walls are much shattered and it trembles with every wind. I think John Quincy Adams will have to move out of it soon. But he himself is quite, quite well!'"

Chapter Five

Questions to Determine If You Are Near the End of Your Life

"When you come near the human race there's layers and layers of nonsense."

Thornton Wilder, *Our Town*

This chapter focuses on questions to ask regarding your diagnosis, time frame and treatment options, all designed to work like a large knife that cuts out the layers of nonsense surrounding the situation. The questions are very direct and courageous; that's exactly what is needed. They are appropriate for new diagnoses and when you need honest, simple answers to plan the remainder of your life.

Tailor these questions to suit your particular situation and add your own before your family conferences with a provider or social worker. Some of the questions are very broad and may not be appropriate to your particular situation. Some may sound strange if it's just for a simple matter like removing a skin cancer or managing a chronic illness that is not life-threatening. These questions emerge from the goals of medicine and the forms of disease in Chapter Three. We begin with simple questions from the ACURE and COPE frameworks. If you were given a terminal diagnosis, you are a CARE individual already, so begin your family conference using that category of questions.

Be aware, too, that chronic illnesses from the COPE form of disease may progress to the CARE form. If a new illness is imposed on top of a chronic ailment, a patient becomes a CARE type. That's called co-morbidity. Think back to the cases of Edwin and Drew. As complication after complication arose, both moved to become CARE patients.

The Interview or Family Conference

For the family conference, bring some of your significant others. Have somebody take notes to record answers to the questions you ask. Select your questions from the lists and form your own well before your family conference. Later on, you and your significant others can discuss the answers. During the family conference, you may be frightened or too anxious to really hear anything at all. If you need more family conferences for other reasons, schedule them as needed. Use the same questions for another provider at a different date. At home, you can compare and contrast the answers.

If you remotely think the treatments offered are futile, use the questions from Chapter Four's "Extraordinary Measures." You have a right to all the information you need to make a true informed decision. Realize, too, that most providers are interested in doing the right thing for you. If you are open, trusting and realistic, they will be honest with you.

These questions may aid you in emerging from the confusion and shock of a life-threatening illness to a place that's clear and positive. After your family conferences, revisit Chapter Three, the goals of medicine and the forms of disease. Please consider the person answering your questions to be on your side.

Let's take a closer look at the groups of questions.

Broad Questions for the First Form of Disease: ACURE (acute, critical, unexpected, responsive, easily diagnosed and treated)

Examples of typical medical problems with ACURE: fracture, laceration, influenza, croup, meningitis, pancreatitis, appendicitis, cataracts, hemorrhoids, nausea, vomiting, indigestion, some sexually transmitted diseases, H. pylori stomach disease, urinary tract obstruction, bowel obstruction, Caesarean section, some skin cancers, fibroid tumors of the uterus.

1. Should I expect a total cure with the treatment you're suggesting?

2. Will this condition and treatment play any role in any future health problems?

3. Will I be hospitalized? How long?

4. When may I return home? When can I return to work?

5. At what intervals must I follow up with you?

6. Will my symptoms disappear after treatment?

7. Will the surgical wound hurt?

8. What alternatives are there to what you suggest?

9. What risks or problems can occur with the treatment you suggest?

Broad Questions for the Second Form of Disease: COPE (chronic, out-patient, palliative, efficacious)

Examples of common medical problems from COPE: chronic pancreatitis, jaundice, eczema, psoriasis, osteoarthritis, rheumatoid arthritis, anemia, obesity, early sarcoidosis, most psychiatric illnesses (neurotic and psychotic), drug abuse, well-controlled diabetes, AIDS, herpes simplex, Epstein-Barr virus, early heart failure, atherosclerosis, coronary heart disease, asthma, early Parkinson's disease, sleep apnea, renal failure, chronic alcoholism, irritable bowel syndrome, ulcerative colitis, Crohn's disease, controlled seizure disorder, early Alzheimer's, early hepatitis B or C, early multiple sclerosis, new stroke, some cancers, chronic obstructive pulmonary disease, hypothyroidism, gout, eating disorders, hypertension, chronic problems of old age.

1. How long will I have this disease?

2. Is there a new cure?

3. How often must I follow up?

4. What must I do to keep it from progressing?

5. Does this disease seem to progress on its own, despite preventative measures I take?

6. What classes, books or help can you provide to slow its pace and soften its effects?

7. How well do the medicines work?

8. What side effects should I expect from any new medications that are prescribed?

9. Can you foresee a time where I may worsen?

10. Could this disease eventually kill me?

11. Are there any treatments or alternatives to the one you are suggesting?

12. If my illness changes over time, will you tell me?

13. Will this disease affect any other organs?

14. Will a consultation with a specialist tell us anything new?

15. Are there any new tests you can order to help better treat me?

16. Do you think I should write an Advance Health Care Directive?

Broad Questions for the Third form of Disease: CARE (critical, active, recalcitrant, eventual)

Examples of medical problems with CARE: Late Alzheimer's Disease, late Parkinson's disease, late drug and alcohol abuse, late starvation and failure to thrive, Stage Four returning cancers of the breast, lungs, liver, bone, brain, pancreas, liver, prostate, colorectal, ovarian, uterine, kidneys and bladder, late hepatitis B and C, cirrhosis of the liver, Huntington's chorea, late multiple sclerosis, late AIDS with complications, late emphysema, late chronic obstructive pulmonary disease, any late stage cardiac disease, late stage respiratory disease, uncontrolled chronic seizure disorders, severe head or chest blunt trauma, severe birth defects, late stage melanomas, uncontrolled diabetes with kidney, cardiac, or osteomyelitis complications (bone infection), morbid obesity, malignant hypertension with stroke or kidney damage, severe spinal cord injury, resistant bacterial infections, Lou Gehrig's Disease (ALS).

The following section is your manual to document the responses from several different providers during the opinion phase. These questions should be used if you were given a terminal diagnosis or are unsure what you were told. Have a family member write down the responses in the spaces provided. You are already a CARE patient if you were given a terminal diagnosis.

1. In your opinion, is there a cure for what I have now?

Opinion One:

Opinion Two:

Opinion Three:

2. Are there any treatments or medicines that can help slow down this disease?

Opinion One:

Opinion Two:

Opinion Three:

3. As this disease progresses, will I experience pain and suffering?

Opinion One:

Opinion Two:

Opinion Three:

4. Where will I experience pain and how severe or frequent will it be in your opinion?

Opinion One:

Opinion Two:

Opinion Three:

5. How will I receive adequate pain relief?

Opinion One:

Opinion Two:

Opinion Three:

6. Will I live to see a cure for this disease?

Opinion One:

Opinion Two:

Opinion Three:

7. Do present treatments hold any promise for me?

Opinion One:

Opinion Two:

Opinion Three:

8. Do present treatments hold more burden or hardship for me?

Opinion One:

Opinion Two:

Opinion Three:

9. Would an experimental treatment or drug benefit me?

Opinion One:

Opinion Two:

Opinion Three:

10. Would you say this disease is now unstoppable?

Opinion One:

Opinion Two:

Opinion Three:

11. Will I eventually die from this disease? If yes, do you have any idea how much more time I have?

Opinion One:

Opinion Two:

Opinion Three:

12. How would you proceed if you or your parent were in my shoes?

Opinion One:

Opinion Two:

Opinion Three:

13. Shall I write my Advance Health Care Directive today?

Opinion One:

Opinion Two:

Opinion Three:

14. Does designating myself as a "do not resuscitate" patient or "no code" patient serve my best interests, considering it will probably take my life?

Opinion One:

Opinion Two:

Opinion Three:

15. Should I prepare a will or trust now (if not already done)?

Opinion One:

Opinion Two:

Opinion Three:

16. Would seeing other specialists extend my life, shorten it or do nothing at all?

Opinion One:

Opinion Two:

Opinion Three:

17. Would having more tests be of any benefit to me now?

Opinion One:

Opinion Two:

Opinion Three:

18. Will you still treat my minor problems like pain, infection, constipation, shortness of breath, anxiety, and feelings of suffocation?

Opinion One:

Opinion Two:

Opinion Three:

19. Will you abandon me if I become too sick to come in anymore?

Opinion One:

Opinion Two:

Opinion Three:

20. Would you say I am in the terminal phase of my disease?

Opinion One:

Opinion Two:

Opinion Three:

21. Are any further medical treatments for me now futile?

Opinion One:

Opinion Two:

Opinion Three:

22. Is it time for me to put my affairs in order?

Opinion One:

Opinion Two:

Opinion Three:

23. Is it okay if I travel by plane, ship, car, train or bus?

Opinion One:

Opinion Two:

Opinion Three:

24. Do I need to return to see you anymore?

Opinion One:

Opinion Two:

Opinion Three:

25. If you think I have less than six months to live, should I enroll in a hospice program today so I can remain at home?

Opinion One:

Opinion Two:

Opinion Three:

26. Can I smoke and drink now?

Opinion One:

Opinion Two:

Opinion Three:

27. Can I eat what I want?

Opinion One:

Opinion Two:

Opinion Three:

28. Can I still have sexual relations?

Opinion One:

Opinion Two:

Opinion Three:

29. Should I still do as much for myself as I can?

Opinion One:

Opinion Two:

Opinion Three:

30. Will this disease cause me to eventually lose my independence?

Opinion One:

Opinion Two:

Opinion Three:

31. Do you have a social work referral to help me navigate through the paperwork and plans for me?

Opinion One:

Opinion Two:

Opinion Three:

32. Should I preplan my funeral now?

Opinion One:

Opinion Two:

Opinion Three:

When I look over these questions and the necessity of being surrounded by loved ones when we must ask them, I'm reminded of a wonderful, comforting comment from 19th Century English novelist George Eliot: "Oh the comfort, the inexpressible comfort of feeling safe with a person; having neither to weigh thoughts or measure words, but to put them all out, just as they are grain and chaff together knowing that a faithful hand will take and sift them, keep what is worth keeping, and then, with the breath of kindness, blow the rest away."

Chapter Six

Your Advance Health Care Directive, the Code Blue, the ICU and a Description of Life on a Breathing Machine

"May you live all the days of your life."
Jonathan Swift, *Gulliver's Travels*

Every state in the United States, plus American territories and commonwealth, has their own versions of the Advance Health Care Directive (AHCD). It may be a good time to obtain one from your clinic, hospital, lawyer's office or download one from the Internet. Usually your state medical association has an up-to-date Advance Health Care Directive kit, which you can download. Your public library may also be of service in helping you obtain a copy today. If you are in California, you may download one by visiting www.cmanet.org.

The California Medical Association has a special kit that you can print out at home. Since I'm a Californian, I'll refer to California's AHCD and discuss all of its important parts. Basically, the sections in the different states' Advance Health Care Directives are the same. Match up what's discussed here to the corresponding section in your home state's Advance Health Care Directive.

Before filling out the AHCD, let's quickly review what you've done before deciding how you'll answer the sections about your personal AHCD regarding life support. I have included a small description in this chapter about what happens during a "code blue" and what life might look like for you or a relative should that happen.

The purpose of the Advance Health Care Directive is to tell paramedics, emergency department staff, your provider, nurses and other staff that you do not or do want CPR, ACLS, life support machines or an extensive stay in the intensive care unit. The choice is simple and clear: either direct all personnel to extend your life for as long as possible, or direct them not to interrupt your peaceful death. This directive should be made if you are identified as a COPE or CARE patient, are elderly or are now in a terminal disease state.

Here are five review questions to ask (there is room to write your responses below):
1. Are you satisfied with your research, family conferences and the opinions you received from your providers, social worker and nurses?

2. Did you identify your particular situation with a form of disease category (ACUTE, COPE, and CARE)?

3. Did you revisit the medical goals for yourself? Which are realistic and doable today?

4. Are your providers and significant others in agreement with what you've decided?

5. Are you all clear about your particular direction?

The other goal of the AHCD is to present a legal document, which you are preparing when you fill out this directive. In California, it becomes a legal document when it is signed by two witnesses who are not your heirs, providers or family members or if signed by a notary public. Be sure to make plenty of copies for yourself, your providers, the hospital and paramedics. Give a copy to your significant others and to the agent you've chosen to speak for you if you can no longer speak for yourself. This can be the executor of your estate or a close family member or friend – someone that will adhere to your wishes, no matter what opposition may exist from others.

If you choose to be a "do not resuscitate" or "no code" patient, it doesn't mean you will be cut off from all care. It's quite the opposite. Everybody will still care for you as before. The only difference is that, if your heart or breathing should stop, you will be allowed a peaceful death with nobody calling the paramedics to perform CPR.

You will be given every comfort care measure, such as nursing care and medicine. You will be positioned to breathe better, you will receive a little oxygen cannula or pipe to wear by your nose, and you will be administered medicine to relieve pain, relax more easily and not be scared. Until the moment of your death, you probably will not be alone, in pain or feeling suffocated. It is a time of "high touch and low tech."

Remember all those "ordinary measures" we discussed before? All those same measures will be performed for you if you designate yourself a "do not resuscitate" or "no code" patient. The only difference is that nobody will interrupt your passing when the moment comes.

For those people who want every measure taken to prolong life, there are a few things to discuss. You have stated your desire to be a "full code," which needs a lot of clarification. A full code is an extraordinary measure for those identified as CARE patients and who were told by their providers that a cure or remission is not possible.

A code blue is a scary and at times violent protocol where providers pound on your chest and insert a large tube through your nose or through your mouth. The tube is connected to a breathing machine. There are no guarantees that your life will be saved during this process, as only about 15% actually survive it. (At the end of this section is a description of the only patient I have known who survived a code blue).

First of all, realize that your providers and hospital staff have no legal, moral or ethical reason to honor your request of remaining as a "full code" if you have a terminal illness and are expected to pass away shortly. A code blue and a life support machine are but band-aids. They offer no cure or remission from a life-threatening disease, especially after it has progressed enough to really threaten your life.

If you survive a code blue, your resulting stay in the intensive care unit may only stop the inevitable for a short time. Once begun, stopping the dying process altogether may prove to be a larger nightmare for you and your family.

Many of the ICU beds are filled with people who did not understand the gravity of their situation, or refused to understand, or whose family could not let go. Many of today's providers are terrified to have that "talk" with their patients and families because of the negative reactions to the thought of death and dying.

What Happens in a Code Blue:
Reader Discretion Advised

You may wish to skip over this next section if you do not want to read about all the "gory" details of a code blue. The purpose of this section is to help you better give informed consent if you wish to have everything possible done to save your life and understand what you will endure.

"Do you want everything done for your loved one?" This is the most frequently asked question when signs of impending death are noted by nurses, providers, and loved ones. But what does "everything" mean exactly?

The following is a raw description of "everything." Cardiopulmonary Resuscitation (CPR) and Advanced Cardiac Life Support (ACLS) are designed to disturb death for previously well people without an incurable illness, or people who were not expected to die. This can include everything from accident victims to athletes who stop breathing on the practice field; the possible scenarios are far too numerous to mention here. Now CPR and ACLS are practiced in all situations and circumstances, even on the very old and those who have an incurable and progressive disease. There are many reasons it is performed: money, fear of being sued, unresolved family issues, fear of death and living in denial. In my opinion, CPR and ACLS should be reserved for trauma victims and for people who were not expected to die. CPR and ACLS, in my opinion, should never be used on people who are expected to pass away in a short time.

Paramedics, emergency medical techs (EMTs), providers in hospital, registered nurses, licensed vocational nurses (LVNs), respiratory therapists and other personnel receive CPR training every year or two, depending on the work setting. Also, teachers, coaches and other employees in public servant positions receive CPR training. Classroom time, demonstration time, and exams are requirements to being certified by the American Heart Association to perform CPR. ACLS has the same requirements, but it involves a longer preparation process of exams, demonstrations and many classes.

If a patient is in respiratory distress, failure or arrest, or if there is a life-threatening heart rhythm, a code blue is usually called in the hospital setting, or on the street if the person has collapsed. If the paramedics arrive on the scene outside the home or if the problem occurs in a hospital setting, a code is called and CPR begins. ACLS takes CPR to a new level with breathing equipment, medicines, and electrical shock. After it is determined that the patient is not breathing, a tube is inserted through the nose or mouth and an airbag squeezed to give the patient a breath. If the heart is in an irregular rhythm, a series of electrical shocks is applied to the chest between chest compressions.

Throughout this process, the team leader follows a pattern in which he or she surveys the patient and shouts out orders to the assembled group. The mantra that guides the process is A-B-C, "airway, breathing, and circulation." The leader assesses each area constantly. Even when a pulse returns, the process still continues if the blood is not circulating on its own. If there are few signs of life after 20 to 30 minutes, the leader may call off the code blue, as brain death has occurred. Brain death arises two to three minutes after the heart stops or does not pump sufficient blood and oxygen to the brain.

The cerebrum needs a constant supply of oxygen and sugar, or it will die in a few minutes. The cerebrum is the seat of your personality. If your cerebrum has died, it is debatable if you are still alive or are a "vegetable," also known as a persistent vegetative state. A person's primitive brain or brain stem may still work: he or she will awaken and sleep at appropriate times, perhaps track movement in the room, and may even look at you. However, the cerebrum or seat of the personality may have already died when the code blue occurred.

What happens afterward is truly an ethical dilemma.

After the code blue, the surviving patient is transported to the intensive care unit (ICU) to receive intensive nursing care. The ratio of specialized ICU registered nurses is two patients per nurse. For the already terminally ill, death has been postponed for a little while. Now a real fool's errand of procedures begins: blood draws several times a day; intensive suctioning and respiratory care by respiratory therapy and nursing; turning and changing often; many diagnostic exams; x-rays; and an assortment of specialists that pass in and out of the room. The ICU hums 24/7. Most cannot tell if it's day or night, as people are serving the patient all the time. Even the lights are on 24/7. You may or may not be conscious, or restrained.

What follows next is a common scenario for those who manage to live for a few days: hospital-borne infections. Because of overuse of antibiotics, we now have strains of bacteria that are totally resistant to everything, even the most effective antibiotics. Hospital-acquired infections are called nosocomial infections; they are pervasive among the population, in schools, prisons, jails, day care centers, nursing homes, clinics and hospitals. Vancomycin resistant enterococcus (VRE) has no known antibiotic that helps; methycillin resistant staphylococcus aureus (MRSA) may soon run out of antibiotics that work. Clostridium difficile (C. diff) may also run out of efficacious antibiotics to kill it.

When you are on life support, have an open wound, a urinary drainage bag, an IV or even a feeding tube surgically inserted in your stomach area, the germs can bypass all natural defenses. If your condition has deteriorated, you may have few defenses left to fight off germs. Local infection soon passes from the skin to the blood, or from the lungs to the blood. Blood-borne bacteria emit chemicals that cause your blood pressure to fall. As the bacteria numbers increase, they emit more chemicals and your blood pressure continues to drop. Now, your ICU nurse needs to normalize your blood pressure with specialized IV drips. Often times, with very low blood pressure, the kidneys will fail and another treatment nightmare sets in: dialysis. Organ failure begins globally, with one organ dysfunction leading to another organ dysfunction – even with the best and most expensive nursing, medical and pharmacy care.

Once on life support, it is difficult to stop this vicious cycle, especially without an Advance Health Care Directive. If your family is directionless, jumpy, scared, fighting, or dependent on your income, they may not want to stop the process and let you go.

Most hospitals have a biomedical ethics committee that, if requested, will provide guidance and support. However, their recommendations are not binding. These ICU scenarios are more common than you may realize.

Remember the code blue survivor whom I referred earlier? Meet Charles, age 48, a truly rare human being who managed to survive *two* code blues. He's the only long-term survivor I have ever met in my 23-year history in health care. Charles was a serious drug abuser who took a lot of methamphetamine, which basically destroyed his left ventricular heart function, leaving the muscle very thick and inefficient. His heart function is very compromised yet, he manages to stay alive.

Charles coded twice in the hospital after a heart attack, both times from an overdose of methamphetamine. He was released to his elderly, widowed mother, also my patient, who has health issues of her own. Charles remains a handsome, trim man. If you looked at him, you would see nothing wrong. He is not in a persistent vegetative state, but has suffered brain damage from the code blues. He smiles appropriately and seems to understand conversation. He will nod his head and say, "yes" or "no" and "thank you" at appropriate intervals.

Otherwise, Charles is quite vacant. Probably, his personality brain cells suffered a loss of oxygen in the minutes before the code; they did not regenerate. He arrives in the kitchen for his meals, ventures to an adult day care center for a few days a week and otherwise spends his days skimming the pool with a large net and pole, over and over. He is also mesmerized by television and sits and watches it all night. Charles becomes agitated constantly, especially if his routine is changed in any way. I see Charles about four times a year and treat him for agitation.

Filling Out the Advance Health Care Directive

By now you should have an Advance Health Care Directive from your state of residence. The first portion answers simple questions in a question-

and-answer format. It is mostly self-explanatory. You will record a list of places and people who will have a copy of your AHCD document.

Next, a section will ask you to appoint your personally designated health care surrogate or agent. Consider that person to be the one who will communicate your wishes if you no longer can – the one person you entrust to carry out all your wishes. There can only be one surrogate or agent at a time, as the position is never shared. The agent's authority stops after death. The agent is not responsible for any of your bills. That is for your estate to settle and your attorney. All property and monies are legal issues for your attorneys to handle, not your providers. Please note that your health insurance cannot deny you benefits if you refuse to make an Advance Health Care Directive or if you make yourself a "do not resuscitate" or "no code" patient or "full code" patient.

How you choose your status as a "full code" or a "do not resuscitate" patient is clearly your personal business. Make your decision without coercion from anybody.

At this point, I'll speak for my parents and myself. If I had a terminal illness and was in the CARE form of the disease, and knowing what I know about disease processes from my experience as a critical care registered nurse and family nurse practitioner, I would choose the "do not resuscitate" approach. I do not fear death – just futile treatments, pain and suffering for no good reason. I do not want to linger in a limbo-land of the ICU, sedated, anesthetized, unable to give or receive love, tied down with restraints, and awakened at all hours for suctioning, turning and having my bottom cleaned. That to me is undignified, a real nightmare and totally against my personal integrity. As for my parents, I would never permit that to occur, especially if they were considered CARE patients with incurable, progressive conditions. What purpose would it serve, considering their ages and disease? Would a wait for an eventual cure be realistic? Would their disease resolve on its own? Not very likely. Besides, what quality of life could they expect?

At this time, I have written out my own added wishes so that each provider will have no wiggle room to order anything futile, or services I do not desire. Part of my directive concerns feeding tubes. There are several varieties of feeding tubes. Before beginning, know that feeding tubes are placed surgically into the stomach or directly into the intestine; some are inserted through the nose, while others pass through a large IV. Total parenteral nutrition (TPN) is administered through a large chest wall type of IV (subclavian central line) or a large tube IV in the arm (PICC line). Feeding tubes run through the nose or abdominal wall (nasogastric tubes, J-tubes or PEG tubes).

The following is my own direction shared word for word, from my Advanced Health Care Directive. It is written in medicalese so there can be no doubt as to what I want.

Optional Instructions

"I am a 'no code' patient. In addition, I do not want feeding tubes (no nasogastric tubes, no TPN, no J-tubes, no PEG tubes). I only desire freedom from anxiety, pain, feelings of suffocation and suffering. If a narcotic hastens my death, so be it, for I know your intention was to relieve my pain and suffering. I thank you in advance. My only desire is nursing comfort measures, positioning, hygiene and help with elimination and only what is considered "ordinary measures." I no longer desire further diagnostics, x-rays, blood draws or chemotherapy. I will take my regular medicines if my providers believe it will enhance my quality of life for today."

Please feel free to add these words to your own health care directive, if that is your wish.

That is the gist of the Advance Health Care Directive. It instructs your desires in plain writing. The Advance Health Care Directive instructs everyone, including your significant others, to try everything to extend your life or to not interrupt your peaceful death. To quote early 20th Century poet Thomas Curtis Clark, "The touch of human hands – not vain, unthinking words, not that cold charity which shuns our misery; We seek a loyal friend who understands and the warmth, the pulsing warmth of human hands."

Chapter Seven

Hospice Is a State of Mind

"That man is a success who has lived well, laughed often and much; who has gained the respect of intelligent men and the love of children; who has filled his niche and accomplished his task; who leaves the world better than he found it, whether by an improved poppy, a perfect poem, or a rescued soul; who never lacked appreciation of earth's beauty or failed to express it; who looked for the best in others and gave the best he had."

Robert Louis Stevenson

During the days of diagnosis and family conferences to make the best plans for yourself and your loved ones, all of you may still hold many fears about the days ahead. It's perfectly natural.

Let's talk about those fears and assign words to them. Internally, you may still feel all those stages of grief as defined by Elisabeth Kubler-Ross. They now have names and aren't wordless, jumbled-up emotions. In addition, you are dealing with your significant others' reaction to grief. Everybody is probably still quite emotional.

Now, let's name the most common fears people face at this crucial time:
The fear of:

- Losing control of bodily functions
- Losing your independence and depending on others to take care of things you can no longer do
- Being a burden on others
- Being confined to a nursing home or hospital bed
- Leaving home
- Nobody visiting you
- Dying alone
- The unknowns
- Pain
- Feeling you can't catch your breath
- Not finding meaning to this phase of your life
- Leaving those you love
- What comes next
- Not making amends with those whom you've hurt and who have hurt you

Despite all that's happened and the cruel twist of fate that seems to have fallen upon you, you are still the same precious human being who makes an impact on those who know you. Even though your physical body has a disease, remember that inside you are whole and intact. You are the same you, not a living, breathing medical diagnosis.

With this knowledge, look again at the world. Doesn't it all take on a new significance? Stop, look and listen to the majesty that surrounds you. This is your earth, stars, sky, trees and birds. This is your moment. In your own way, be grateful for the gift of life and the fact you have tasted it all: nature, the love of others and the privilege of loving them. That is my definition of what it means to be alive. Maybe now you will have the ability to toss away your cares and see this wonderful world in all its majesty. This is your time, your space; make it special! Even though it may be just for a little while, live the rest of your life well, with grace, composure and dignity.

Now that the hard work is done, you have knowledge of where you are, understand the form of disease called CARE and the appropriate medical goals of medicine. Let's talk about your options that will help dispel your very real fears.

Hospice or palliative care is not a particular place or an address. It is a state of mind and a holistic form of care. Hospice can take place in your house, your living room or bedroom. Hospice also can be a health care facility like a hospital or skilled nursing home. You don't have to leave your home; you can stay put without ever returning to the hospital again. Your life at home will be the same; your friends and family will know where you are. You can eat the same foods you like, drink the same beverages, watch your own TV programs and use your own bathroom.

With your enrollment in a hospice program, your hospice care giver will call on you and step up care in areas that you require. Your hospice care workers will provide you with a high level of comfort care: freedom from pain, isolation, anxiety, and feelings of suffocation. They will give you all those "ordinary measures" discussed in previous chapters. They will manage any short-term problems like infection, wound care, shortness of breath, constipation and problems associated with immobility. They will attempt to keep you as comfortable as possible until you pass away at home, in your own environment.

Hospice involves a multidisciplinary team: nurses, a doctor, housekeepers, social workers, clergy, therapists and assorted volunteers. Your family may also become involved in your care at home. Hospice also establishes support for your family before and after you pass away.

Outside of the hospice setting, many providers are scared to use narcotics, for many reasons. In hospice, the overriding goal is to keep you comfortable, to relieve anxiety and feelings of suffocation. That is its intention. A consequence of narcotics is to depress your effort to breathe. Narcotics in the hospice setting are used judiciously with the intention to keep you comfortable, and never to hasten death. The intention alone is worthy, ethical and legal.

Depending on location, many hospices may include a health care facility that can provide both in-patient and out-patient care. Some people enter the hospice care facility and remain there until their natural deaths. Some go there to provide a rest for their care givers for a few days, and then are transferred back home. The in-house hospice center also can provide better pain control and IVs for hydration. After stabilization, the patient returns back home with the same hospice workers. If, for any reason, your management at home is not working out, your hospice worker will transfer you to the in-patient hospice care center, where you can remain with the same level of care. Whether you receive your hospice care in-patient or at home, you will get the same compassionate service.

Another important aspect to hospice is its spiritual care. Clergy are on staff and you may have your own rabbi, clergyman, priest or imam call on you at home or in the hospice care center. Prayers and religious services also can be arranged for you wherever you desire. All you have to do is ask.

The idea of hospice is relatively new in the United States. In the 1940's, Dr. Cicely Saunders founded St. Christopher Hospice in London, England. It was named for St. Christopher, the patron saint of travelers and pilgrims. Dr. Saunders' hospice was so successful that she was invited to the United States to lecture at Yale University School of Nursing in 1964. Dr. Saunders' philosophy of hospice resounds in modern hospices today all over the world: healing, not curing; ultimate comfort; and freedom from pain and suffering. Hospice is totally focused on your immediate physical and spiritual needs. Hospice workers focus on you retaining your dignity, alertness and sense of control. There are no games or fool's errands. Hospice's goal is making every day count for you, without reservation.

If you want to enroll in a hospice program, the process is very easy. Your health care provider will make the referral. Usually within one working day, a social worker will come to your home or hospital and enroll you. To enroll, you must meet these two criteria:

1. You must be a CARE patient with less than six months to live;

2. You must have an Advance Health Care Directive stating you are a "do not resuscitate" or "no code" patient.

Hospice's goal is not to interrupt a peaceful death. Hospice is your last health care stop. You will receive the highest quality, highest comfort care so you can live out your final days and pass away at home. Hospice will evaporate most of your fears and your family's fears.

When I went to Antarctica in January 2008, we stopped in the southernmost city on the planet, Ushuaia, which sits at the foot of Tierra del Fuego in Argentina. As the cruise ship pulled into majestic Beagle Bay, I was awed by the snow-capped Andes Mountains, the sub-alpine pastures, the tree line, the chalets and sparkling calm ocean in full sunshine. It was a gorgeous day! But what truly took my breath away was a sign in English, in large letters greeting all the ships: "Ushuaia, Argentina, the end of the world and the beginning of everything."

The Hospice Experience of Rose

Rose, age 63, was my patient for about three years. She was a petite woman, well-dressed, coiffed and elegant, with perfect nails and make-up. Over time, due to advanced alcoholism, she was losing weight. Chardonnay over ice was her favorite beverage; she drank it while holding a cigarette like Bette Davis, her favorite pose. Initially, Rose was able to hold down a job as a realtor and never appeared drunk in public. Over the next three years, her weight plummeted from 112 pounds to 72 pounds.

Like many people, Rose had neither health insurance nor any savings. Due to her economic situation, I rarely could get labs and never a chest x-ray. In the clinic, I could administer a urinalysis; early on, I noted she was in ketosis, using up her muscle mass for protein and energy – which happens in cases of starvation. The alcohol and poor nutrition were cause for the weight loss and concern.

As her addiction advanced, Rose consumed mostly alcohol and no longer confined her drinking to the hours after five o'clock. Now she was drinking day and night. The insufficient amount of protein, carbohydrate and calories caused her body to be weak and very thin. The starvation component actually was more alarming than the alcoholism.

At every turn, I advised Rose to stop drinking and to treat her underlying depression and anxiety. She took the prescriptions but never filled them. Her daughter even made a reservation in a rehab detoxification center and offered to pay for a three-month in-patient stay. Rose declined.

In a few months, Rose was unemployed. She was unable to stand for long periods, becoming shaky if she didn't get a drink after a few hours. Soon she looked like an Auschwitz survivor – emaciated, pale and unkempt. I visited her home to have the "talk." Since the alcoholism and starvation were so advanced and she would not stop drinking, I wanted to enroll her in a hospice program, and obtain her emergency county health insurance and her social security retirement early. Rose agreed.

The next day, the social worker for our local hospice called on Rose, enrolled her and completed the paperwork. All the other systems kicked in right away: social security checks and emergency county health insurance to pay for hospice. Rose loved the program and her multidisciplinary team. The volunteers did a lot to help her, including light housekeeping, laundry, and other errands. Her nurses were wonderful to her and she delighted in their visits.

Throughout her hospice care, she increased her addiction to chardonnay until she was drinking day and night and no longer eating much. She was very wasted now, nearing 72 pounds. Before long, she was using a walker but had enough strength to get from her sofa to bed to the toilet on her own. The funniest irony was Rose's choice of TV programs; they were on the *cooking* and *food* channels. She wrote out elaborate recipes and told us what she'd be cooking; eventually, she created exquisite dishes for everybody else to eat. In all, Rose was stable with the in-home hospice.

After about five months, she called me quite late one evening to visit right away. She was in bed, completely incontinent. So I changed her, then the bed sheets. When I arrived at her home, her pulse was very high and she had a fever. I called in hospice, as Rose was talking gibberish, her words like a tossed salad. Before long, she was transferred to the in-house hospice when I suspected dehydration and a urinary tract infection.

Rose lasted one more week; she never returned to her apartment. I visited her at the hospice care center where I found her outside in the patio with her daughter, smoking a cigarette and holding a glass of icy chardonnay. On the following Sunday morning, hospice called to say Rose had passed away in her sleep.

The hospice referral fulfilled Rose's wishes perfectly: she got to stay at home until a week before she died; she could drink and smoke as she pleased; and she was safe at home because the care workers visited her daily. When she became too unstable and at risk of her own safety, they correctly stepped up the care. Until the end, Rose stated she had no pain, anxiety or feelings of suffocation. According to her daughter, Rose had very happy moments while she visited her. Rose had it all her way.

Chapter Eight

Conclusion and Going Forward

After Benjamin Franklin had received a letter thanking him for having done a kindness, he replied: "As to the kindness you mention, I wish I could have been of more service to you than I have been, but if I had, the only thanks that I should desire are that you would always be ready to serve any other person that may need your assistance, and so let offices go around, for mankind are all of a family. As for my own part, when I am employed in serving others I do not look upon myself as conferring favors but paying debts."

Thank you for permitting me to be your doting godfather, your trustworthy old friend and your battle-scarred nurse. Thank you for listening to my stories. I hope my little gift of this book will provide you a measure of sanity, well-being and comfort. This gift also comes from all the people I cared for, who gave me their gifts to pass along. They have given me more than what I did for them. So goes the circle of debt repayment.

Sometimes, when I look out at my surroundings and the majesty of the earth and stars, I feel sometimes that all the people I served are looking out through my eyes, too. Sometimes I imagine their memory propels me forward to offer small gifts to others, and now to you. I guess that giving away my abundance has been my lot in life and my greatest joy, even as a little boy. Really, it seems like a charmed life of generosity and grace, connectedness and care. It feels like I win the jackpot everyday!

At times, *Sooner or Later* was hard to write; at others, I found my pen had a mind of its own. I felt for you, struggling with all that emotion and information that brought its own harsh realities. I guess our pilgrimage as human beings is just a balancing act of walking on a tightrope, trying to balance the truly awesome with the truly terrifying.

I hope you may begin to find your way with this small roadmap. I hope some of your questions were answered and you are not afraid. By now, you know where all the answers lie: in the deep well-spring that is uniquely you. You never really needed to look any further than your own backyard. Now click your heels three times and exclaim as Dorothy did in *The Wizard of Oz*, "There's no place like home! There's no place like home! There's no place like home!"

Success

To laugh often and love much,
To win the respect of intelligent people and the
affection of children,
To earn the appreciation of honest critics and
endure the betrayal of false friends,
To appreciate beauty,
To find the best in others,
To give of one's self,
To leave the world a little better, whether by a
healthy child, a garden patch,
or a redeemed social condition,
To have played and laughed with enthusiasm
and sung with exultation,
To know even one life breathed easier,
This is to have succeeded.

Ralph Waldo Emerson

About the Author

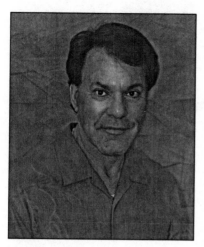

Damiano de Sano Iocovozzi, MSN FNP CNS is a world traveler, linguist and family nurse practitioner. From an early age, growing up in upstate New York, he was fascinated with languages, the spirit of giving and knowledge of other cultures and countries. Damiano completed years of language study and work in Italy, France and Germany. Later, he became a Peace Corps Volunteer and served in a small high school in Meknes, Morocco.

After the Peace Corps, Damiano traveled to San Francisco, California where he worked as an international tour director, leading organized tours around the world. However, Damiano found his true calling becoming a registered nurse and clinical nurse specialist upon earning his degree from the University of San Francisco. During the AIDS epidemic, he specialized in caring for the very sick on a local AIDS hospital floor.

Damiano completed a post-Master's certificate as a family nurse practitioner from Samuel Merritt College where he worked as an instructor for nine years. He also worked as a clinical nurse specialist and educator for Summit Hospital in Oakland. He served veterans as a family nurse practitioner for a number of years in Vallejo, California. Damiano worked in a number of small clinics in primary care and cardiology in Palm Springs, California, where he currently lives.

www.SoonerorLaterBook.com

Bibliography

Jonsen A., Siegler M., Winslade W., (1986). *Clinical Ethics.* Macmillan Publishing Company, New York

Kubler-Ross, E. (1969) *On Death and Dying,* Macmillan Publishing Company, New York

Additional Notes